Simple Keto Vegetarian Recipes

Lose Weight and Feel Great with these Delicious and Easy to Prepare Plant-Based Ketogenic Recipes

Lidia Wong

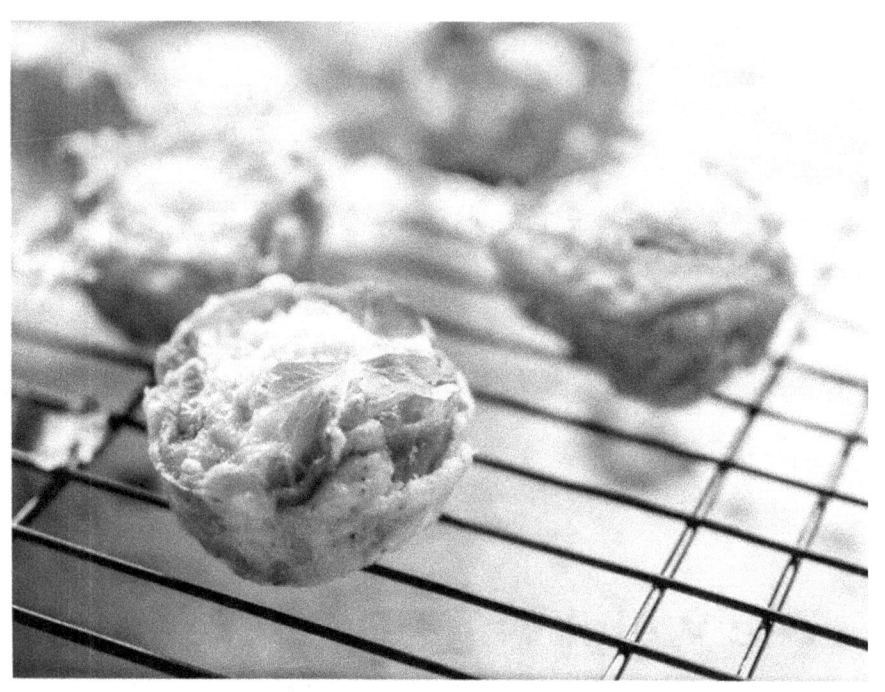

© **Copyright 2021 by Lidia Wong - All rights reserved.**

The content contained within this book may not be reproduced, duplicated or transmitted without direct written permission from the author or the publisher.
Under no circumstances will any blame or legal responsibility be held against the publisher, or author, for any damages, reparation, or monetary loss due to the information contained within this book. Either directly or indirectly.

Legal Notice:
This book is copyright protected. This book is only for personal use. You cannot amend, distribute, sell, use, quote or paraphrase any part, or the content within this book, without the consent of the author or publisher.

Disclaimer Notice:
Please note the information contained within this document is for educational and entertainment purposes only. All effort has been executed to present accurate, up to date, and reliable, complete information. No warranties of any kind are declared or implied. Readers acknowledge that the author is not engaging in the rendering of legal, financial, medical or professional advice. The content within this book has been derived from various sources. Please consult a licensed professional before attempting any techniques outlined in this book.
By reading this document, the reader agrees that under no circumstances is the author responsible for any losses, direct or indirect, which are incurred as a result of the use of information contained within this document, including, but not limited to, — errors, omissions, or inaccuracies.

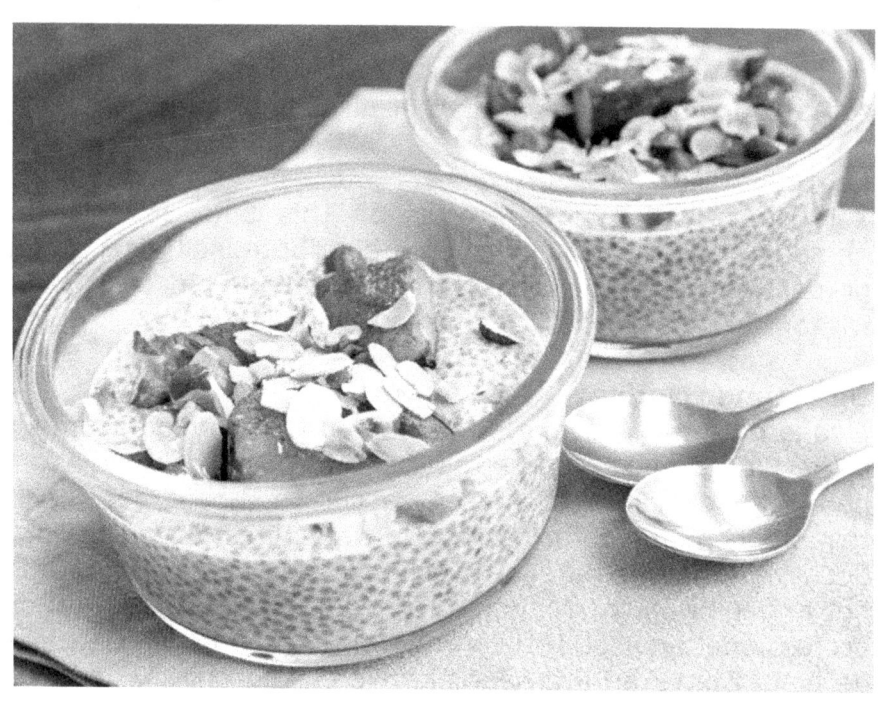

TABLE OF CONTENTS

INTRODUCTION 1

Coconut Pecan Porridge 3

Bulletproof Coffee 5

Creamy Brussels Sprouts Bowls 6

Fruity Cauliflower Rice Bowls 8

Spicy Asian Broccoli 9

Tofu Scramble 11

Roasted Green Beans 13

Caramelized Endive with Garlic 15

Curried Cauliflower Mash 16

Simple Roasted Radishes 18

Green Parsley Broccoli Cauliflower Puree 20

Simple Cheese olives Tomato Salad 22

Seitan Cauliflower Bowl 23

Cajun Tofu in Mushrooms 25

Stewed Tofu with Walnut Cauliflower Grits 27

Tempeh Mushroom Omelet 30

Tempeh Coconut Curry Bake 32

Tempeh Garam Masala Bake 34

Jalapeno Zucchinis Mix	36
Creamy Eggplant Mix	37
Chives Kale and Tomato	39
Ginger Mushrooms	41
Basil Green Beans	43
Cauliflower and Chives Mash	45
Crispy Zucchini Fries	47
Cajun Sweet Potatoes	50
Miso Spaghetti Squash	52
Baked Potatoes and "BBQ" Lentils	54
Fresh Fruit Smoothie	56
Green Vegetable Smoothie	58
Celery Stew	59
Sautéed Mustard Greens	61
Roasted Asparagus	63
Arugula and Broccoli Soup	65
Basil Tomato Soup	67
Black Bean Soup With A Splash	69
Coconut Tofu Zucchini Bake	71
Creamy Avocado-Dressed Kale Salad	73
Classic Potato Salad	76
Garden Salad Wraps	78

Almond Lemon Biscuits 80

Zesty Orange-Cranberry Energy Bites 82

Pumpkin Spice Cake 84

Peanut Butter & Chocolate Cheesecake 86

Chocolate Bread Pudding. 88

Cheesecake 90

Berry Cake 92

Cinnamon Avocado and Berries Mix 94

Chocolate Pudding 95

Grapes Pie 97

Walnuts Cream 98

Chia & Coco Shake (vegan) 99

NOTE **101**

INTRODUCTION

The keto diet is the shortened term for ketogenic diet and it is essentially a high-fat and low-carb diet that helps you lose weight, thereby bringing various health benefits. This diet drastically restricts your carb intake while increasing your fat intake; this pushes your body to go into a state know as "*ketosis*". We will tackle ketosis in a bit.

The human body uses glucose from carbs to fuel metabolic pathways—meaning various bodily functions like digestion, breathing, etc.. Essentially, anything that needs energy. Even when you are resting, the body needs fuel or energy for you to continue living. If you think about it, when have you ever stopped breathing, or your heart stopped beating, or your liver stopped from cleansing the body, or your kidneys from filtering blood?

Never, unless you're dead, which is the only time in which the body doesn't need energy. In normal circumstances, glucose is the primary pathway when it comes to sourcing the body's energy.

But the body also has another pathway; it can utilize fats to fuel the various bodily processes. And this is what we call "*ketosis*". And the body can only enter ketosis when there is no glucose available, thus the reason for sticking to a low-carb diet is essential in the keto diet. Since no glucose is available, the body is pushed to use fats—it can either come from the food you consume or from your body's fat reserves—the adipose tissue or from the flabby parts of your body. This is how the keto diet helps you lose weight, by burning up all those stored fats that you have and using it to fuel bodily processes.

That said, if for whatever reason you are a vegetarian, following a ketogenic diet can be extremely difficult. A vegetarian diet is largely free of animal products, which means that food tends to be usually high in carbohydrates. Still, with careful planning, it is possible. This Cookbook will provide you with various easy and delicious dishes to help you stick to your ketogenic diet plan while being a vegetarian.

Enjoy!

Coconut Pecan Porridge

Preparation Time: 5 minutes

Cooking Time: 5 minutes

Servings: 2

Ingredients:

- ½ teaspoon cinnamon
- ¼ cup pecans, chopped
- 2 tablespoons chia seeds
- ¼ cup coconut, unsweetened, toasted
- ¼ cup coconut milk
- ¾ cup almond milk, unsweetened
- 1 tablespoon coconut oil
- 2 tablespoons hemp seeds
- ¼ cup almond butter

Directions:

1. Add almond butter, coconut oil, almond milk, coconut milk into a saucepan and simmer over medium heat for 5 minutes or so.

2. Once your mixture has reached the point of becoming hot, remove it from heat.
3. Add toasted coconut, hemp seeds, chia seeds, cinnamon, and pecans, mix well.
4. Set aside for 5 minutes.
5. Serve and enjoy!

Nutritional Values (Per Serving):

Calories: 489 Fat: 47.9 g Carbohydrates: 15.1 g
Sugar: 3.9 g Protein: 11.2 g Cholesterol: 0 mg

Bulletproof Coffee

Preparation Time: 3 minutes

Serving: 2

Ingredients:

- 2 ½ heaping tbsp. ground bulletproof coffee beans
- 1 cup water
- 1 tbsp MCT oil
- 2 tbsp unsalted butter

Directions:

1. Using a coffee maker, brew one cup of coffee with the ground coffee beans and water.
2. Transfer the coffee to a blender and add the MCT oil and butter. Blend the mixture until frothy and smooth.
3. Divide the drink into two teacups and enjoy it immediately.

Nutrition:

Calories:64, Total Fat:7.3 g, Saturated Fat: 5.3g, Total Carbs:3 g, Dietary Fiber: 2g, Sugar: 2g, Protein: 3g, Sodium: 300mg

Creamy Brussels Sprouts Bowls

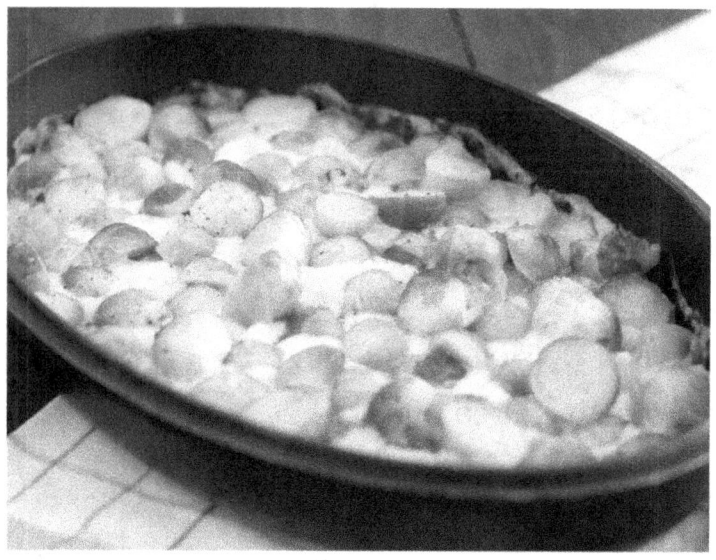

Preparation time: 10 minutes

Cooking time: 30 minutes

Servings: 4

Ingredients:

- 1-pound Brussels sprouts, trimmed and halved
- 1 tablespoon olive oil
- 1 cup coconut cream
- ½ teaspoon chili powder
- ½ teaspoon garam masala

- ½ teaspoon garlic powder
- A pinch of salt and black pepper
- 1 tablespoon lime juice

Directions:

1. In a roasting pan, combine the sprouts with the cream, chili powder and the other ingredients, toss, introduce in the oven at 380 degrees F and bake for 30 minutes.
2. Divide into bowls and serve for lunch.

Nutrition:

calories 219, fat 18.3, fiber 5.7, carbs 14.1, protein 5.4

Fruity Cauliflower Rice Bowls

Preparation time: 10 minutes

Cooking time: 0 minutes

Servings: 4

Ingredients:

- ½ cup grapes, halved
- ½ cup blackberries, halved
- 2 cups cauliflower rice, steamed
- 1 cup cherry tomatoes, halved
- 1 avocado, peeled, pitted and cubed
- 2 tablespoons avocado oil
- Juice of 1 lime

Directions:

1. In a salad bowl, combine the cauliflower rice with the berries and the other ingredients, toss, divide into smaller bowls and serve.

Nutrition:

calories 138, fat 10.9, fiber 5.3, carbs 11.1, protein 1.8

Spicy Asian Broccoli

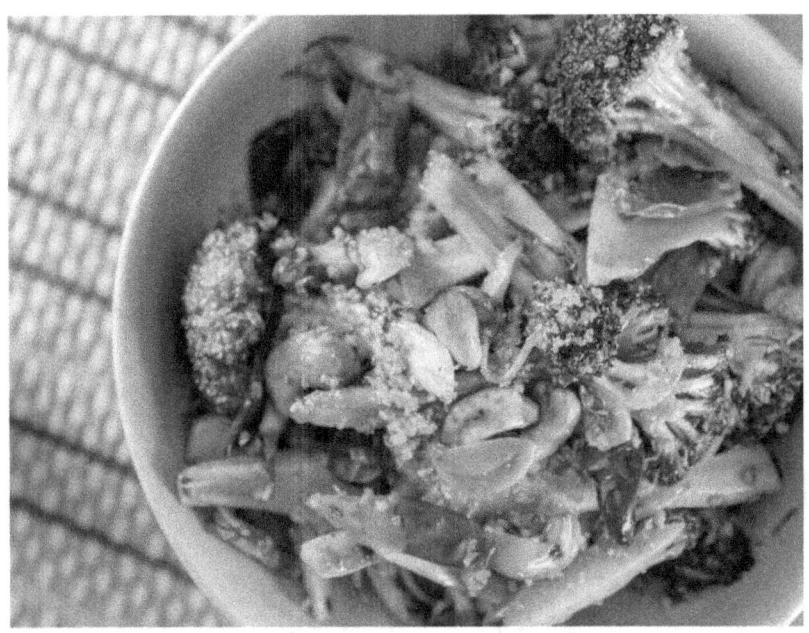

Preparation Time: 25 minutes

Cooking Time: 8 minutes

Servings: 4

Ingredients:

- 2 small broccoli, cut into florets
- 2 teaspoon chili pepper, chopped
- 2 fresh limes' juice
- 2 tablespoons ginger, fresh, grated

- 4 garlic cloves, chopped
- 8 tablespoons olive oil

Directions:

1. Add your broccoli florets into your steamer and steam them for 8 minutes.
2. Meanwhile, to prepare dressing, add lime juice, garlic, chili pepper, oil, and ginger in a small mixing bowl and combine.
3. Add steamed broccoli in a large mixing bowl and drizzle over it the dressing.
4. Toss to blend.
5. Serve and enjoy!

Nutritional Values (Per Servings):

Calories: 294 Fat: 26.6 g Carbohydrates: 9.4 g Sugar: 3.2 g Protein: 6.3 g Cholesterol: 0 mg

Tofu Scramble

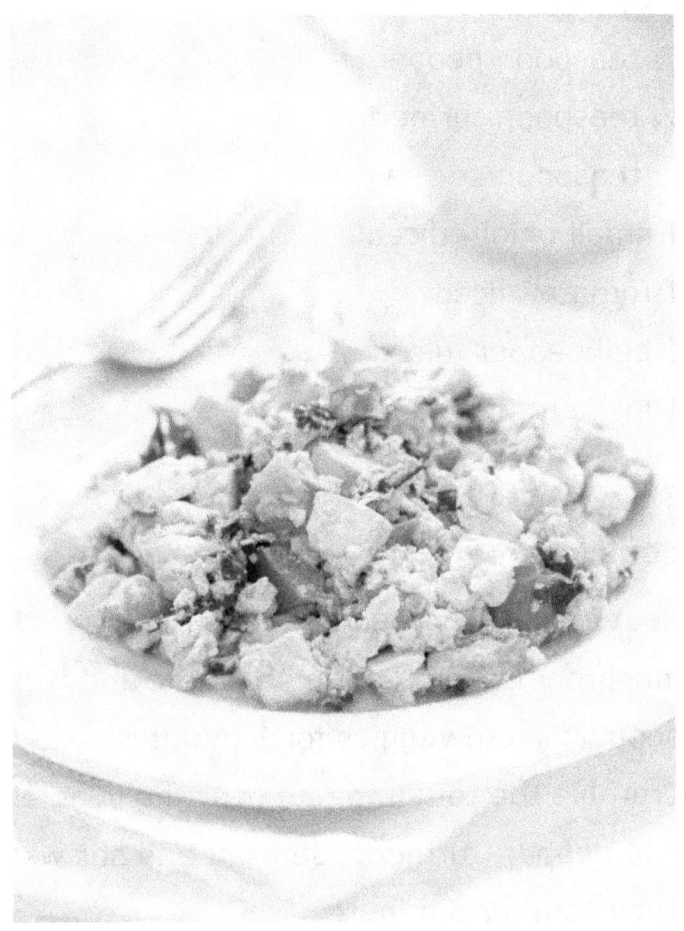

Preparation Time: 10 minutes

Cooking Time: 10 minutes

Servings: 4

Ingredients:

- 1 garlic clove, minced
- 1 cup mushrooms, sliced
- ½ teaspoon pepper
- ½ teaspoon turmeric
- ½ teaspoon sea salt
- 1 small onion, diced
- 1 tomato, diced
- 1 bell pepper, diced
- 1 lb. tofu, firm, drained

Directions:

1. Heat a pan over medium heat, adding mushrooms, tomato, onion, garlic and bell pepper, sauté veggies for 5 minutes.
2. Crumble the tofu into pan over the veggies.
3. Add pepper, turmeric, sea salt and stir well.
4. Cook tofu for 5 minutes.
5. Serve and enjoy!

Nutritional Values (Per Serving):

Calories: 105 Cholesterol: 0mg Sugar: 3.7 g Fat: 5 g Carbohydrates: 7.6 g Protein: 10.6 g

Roasted Green Beans

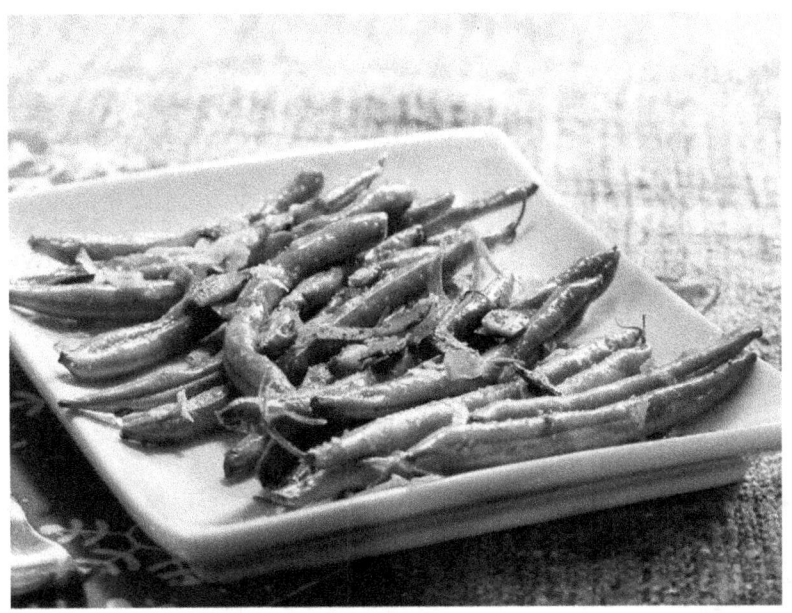

Preparation Time: 15 minutes

Cooking Time: 30 minutes

Servings: 4

Ingredients:

- 1 lb. green beans, frozen
- ½ teaspoon onion powder
- 2 tablespoons extra-virgin olive oil
- ½ teaspoon garlic powder

- ½ teaspoon sea salt
- ½ teaspoon pepper

Directions:

1. Preheat your oven to 425°Fahrenheit. Spray a cooking tray with cooking spray.
2. In a bowl, add all your ingredients and mix well.
3. Spread the green beans on the prepared baking tray and bake for 30 minutes.
4. Serve and enjoy!

Nutritional Values (Per Serving):

Calories: 98 Sugar: 1.8 g Carbohydrates: 8.8 g Fat: 7.2 g Cholesterol: 0 mg Protein: 2.2 g

Caramelized Endive with Garlic

Preparation Time: 10 minutes

Cooking Time: 22 minutes

Servings: 8

Ingredients:

- 2 tablespoons shallots, sliced
- 1 teaspoon garlic, chopped
- 4 heads endive, sliced in half
- ¼ teaspoon pepper
- ¼ cup coconut oil
- ½ teaspoon sea salt

Directions:

1. Melt the coconut oil in a pan over low heat. Once it has melted add shallots, and garlic and cook for 2 minutes.
2. Place endive in the pan and cook for 20 minutes on low heat. Season with salt and pepper.
3. Serve and enjoy!

Nutritional Values (Per Serving):

Calories: 105 Cholesterol: 0 mg Sugar: 0.6 g Fat: 7.3 g Carbohydrates: 9.2 g Protein: 3.3 g

Curried Cauliflower Mash

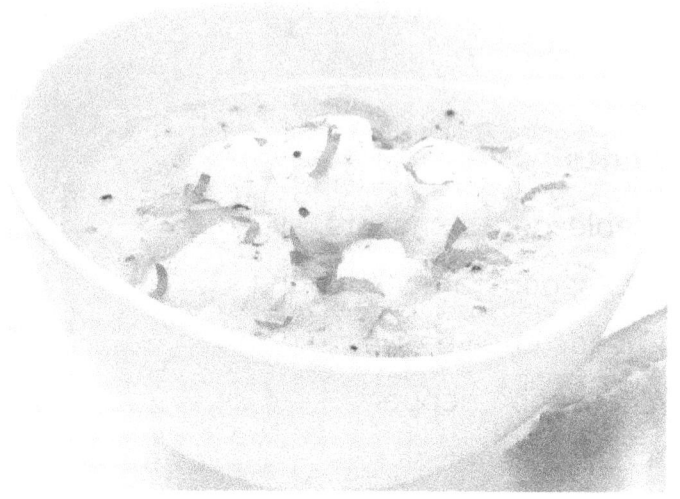

Preparation Time: 10 min

Cooking Time: 10 min

Serves: 4

Ingredients:

- 400 grams Cauliflower
- ½ cup Coconut Milk
- 1 liter Vegetable Stock
- 2 tbsp Curry Powder
- 2 tbsp Tamari

Directions:

1. Bring vegetable stock to a boil in a pot.
2. Add cauliflower and simmer until fully tender and all the stock has evaporated.
3. Stir in coconut milk, curry, and tamari.
4. Puree with an immersion blender.
5. Simmer for 1-2 minutes or until slightly thick.
6. Season with salt as needed.

Nutritional Values:

Kcal per serve: 110 Fat: 8 g. Protein: 4 g. Carbs: 8 g.

Simple Roasted Radishes

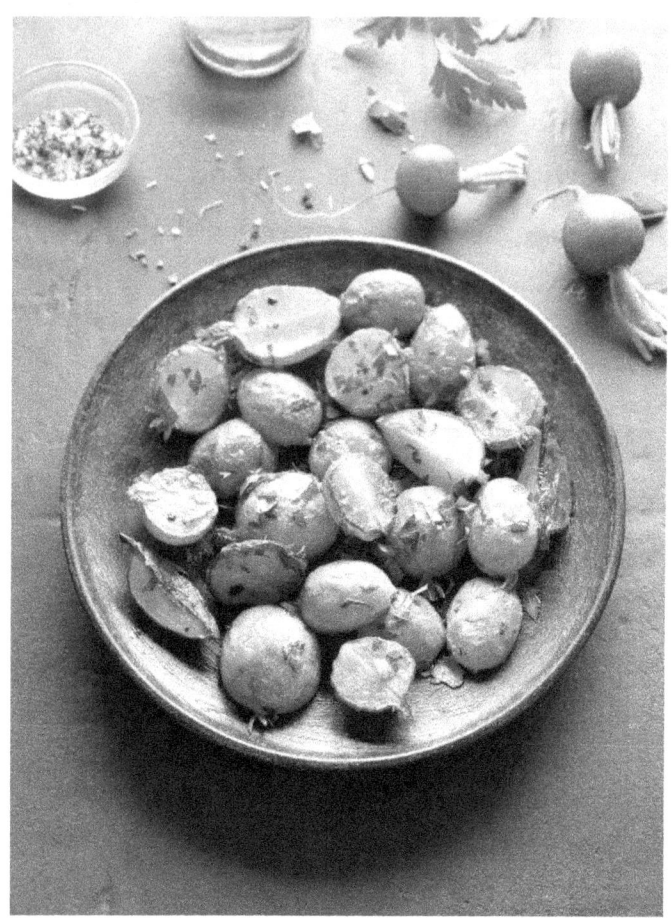

Preparation Time: 45 minutes

Servings: 2

Ingredients:

- 3 cups radish, clean and halved
- 3 tbsp olive oil
- 2 tbsp fresh rosemary, chopped
- 10 black peppercorns, crushed
- 2 tsp sea salt

Directions:

1. Preheat the oven to 425 °F.
2. Add radishes, salt, peppercorns, rosemary, and 2 tablespoons of olive oil in a bowl and toss well.
3. Pour the radishes mixture into the baking sheet and bake in preheated oven for 30 minutes.
4. Heat remaining olive oil in a pan over medium heat.
5. Add baked radishes in the pan and sauté for 2 minutes.
6. Serve immediately and enjoy.

Nutritional Value (Amount per Serving):

Calories 220 Fat 21 g Carbohydrates 8 g Sugar 3 g Protein 1 g Cholesterol 0 mg

Green Parsley Broccoli Cauliflower Puree

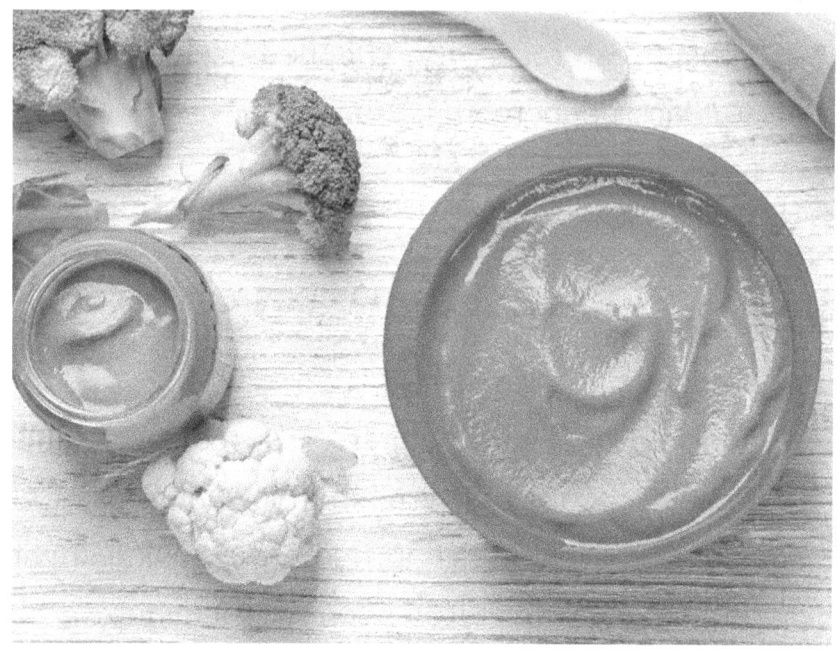

Preparation Time: 35 minutes

Servings: 4

Ingredients:

- 1 1/3 small broccoli, cut into florets
- 1 small cauliflower, cut into florets
- 4 tbsp fresh parsley
- 2 cups vegetable broth

- 4 tbsp butter
- 1 tsp sea salt

Directions:

1. Add cauliflower and broccoli in steamer and steam for 15 minutes.
2. Add steamed cauliflower and broccoli in a blender with butter, broth, and parsley and blend until smooth.
3. Season puree with salt and serve.

Nutritional Value (Amount per Serving):

Calories 154 Fat 12 g Carbohydrates 7 g Sugar 2 g Protein 5 g Cholesterol 31 mg

Simple Cheese olives Tomato Salad

Preparation Time: 15 minutes

Servings: 4

Ingredients:

- 1 cup kalamata olives, pitted
- 1 cup cherry tomatoes, halved
- 1 cup mozzarella cheese, chopped
- Pepper
- Salt

Directions:

1. Add olives, cheese, and tomatoes in a bowl and toss well.
2. Season with pepper and salt.
3. Serve and enjoy.

Nutritional Value (Amount per Serving):

Calories 67 Fat 5 g Carbohydrates 4 g Sugar 1 g Protein 2 g Cholesterol 4 mg

Seitan Cauliflower Bowl

Preparation Time: 10 minutes

Cooking Time: 22 minutes + 1 hour marinating

Servings: 4

Ingredients:

- 4 large eggs
- ¼ cup coconut aminos
- ½ lemon, juiced
- 3 tsp garlic powder
- 1 cup olive oil
- 1 tbsp swerve sugar
- 1 lb seitan, cut into strips
- 6 garlic cloves, minced
- 2 ½ cups cauliflower rice
- 2 tbsp olive oil
- 2 tbsp chopped fresh scallions, for garnishing

Directions:

1. In a medium bowl, mix the coconut aminos, lemon juice, garlic powder, and swerve sugar.
2. Add the seitan, coat well in the mix and

marinate for 1 hour.

3. Heat the olive oil in a medium wok and fry the seitan on both sides until brown and cooked through, 10 minutes. Transfer the seitan to a plate and set aside for serving.
4. Sauté the garlic in the wok until fragrant, 30 seconds. Stir in the cauliflower rice until softened, 5 minutes and season with salt and black pepper. Spoon the food into 4 serving bowls and set aside.
5. Wipe the wok clean with a paper towel and heat in 1 tablespoon of olive oil.
6. Crack in two eggs and fry sunshine-style, 1 minute. Place an egg on each cauliflower rice bowl and fry the remaining eggs with the remaining olive oil. Plate also.
7. Divide the seitan on the food, garnish with some scallions, and serve immediately.

Nutrition:

Calories:823, Total Fat: 75.5g, Saturated Fat:14 g, Total Carbs: 8 g, Dietary Fiber: 2g, Sugar:2 g, Protein: 31g, Sodium: 198mg

Cajun Tofu in Mushrooms

Preparation Time: 10 minutes

Cooking Time: 43 minutes

Serving: 4

Ingredients:

- 2 tbsp olive oil
- ½ celery stalk, chopped
- 1 small red onion, finely chopped
- 1 lb tofu, pressed and crumbled
- 2 tbsp mayonnaise
- 4 large caps Portobello mushrooms
- 1 tsp Cajun seasoning
- ½ tsp garlic powder
- ½ cup shredded Gouda cheese
- 2 large eggs
- Salt and black pepper to taste
- 1 tbsp almond meal
- 2 tbsp shredded Parmesan cheese
- 1 tbsp chopped fresh parsley

Directions:

1. Preheat the oven to 350 °F and lightly grease a baking sheet with cooking spray. Set aside.

2. Heat half of the olive oil in a medium skillet over medium heat and sauté the celery, red onion until softened, 3 minutes. Transfer to a medium mixing bowl.
3. Add the remaining olive oil to the skillet, season the tofu with salt, black pepper, and cook until brown, 10 minutes. Turn the heat off and transfer to the same bowl.
4. Pour in the mayonnaise, Cajun seasoning, garlic powder, Gouda cheese, and crack in the eggs. Mix well.
5. Arrange the mushrooms on the baking sheet and fill with the tofu mix.
6. In a small bowl, mix the almond meal, Parmesan cheese, and sprinkle on top of the mushroom filling. Cover with foil and bake in the oven until the cheese melts, 30 minutes.
7. Remove the stuffed mushrooms, take off the foil, and garnish with the parsley.
8. Serve immediately.

Nutrition:

Calories: 400, Total Fat: 29.1g, Saturated Fat: 8.1g, Total Carbs: 10 g, Dietary Fiber:3 g, Sugar: 2g, Protein:29 g, Sodium: 414mg

Stewed Tofu with Walnut Cauliflower Grits

Preparation Time: 15 minutes

Cooking Time: 53 minutes

Serving: 4

Ingredients:

For the stewed tofu:

- 2 tbsp olive oil
- 2 lb tofu, cut into 1-inch cubes
- 1 large yellow onion, chopped
- 3 garlic cloves, minced
- 2 large tomatoes, diced
- Salt and black pepper to taste
- 1 tbsp rosemary
- 1 tbsp smoked paprika
- 2 tsp chili powder
- 2 cups vegetable broth

For the walnut cauliflower grits:

- 2 tbsp butter
- ½ cup walnuts, chopped

- 2 cups cauliflower rice
- 1 cup coconut milk
- ½ cup water
- 1 cup shredded provolone cheese
- Salt to taste

Directions:

For the stewed tofu:

1. Heat the olive oil in a large pot over medium heat, season the tofu with salt and black pepper and cook in the oil until brown, 3 minutes.
2. Stir in the remaining ingredients and cook over low heat until thickened, 5 to 10 minutes.
3. Adjust the taste with salt and black pepper, and turn the heat off.

For the walnut cauliflower grits:

4. Melt the butter in a medium pot and toast in the walnuts for 5 minutes.
5. Transfer to a cutting board, chop and reserve in a plate.
6. Add the cauliflower rice and water to the pot and cook for 5 minutes or until softened.

7. Stir in the coconut milk, reduce the temperature, and simmer for 3 minutes.
8. Mix in the provolone cheese to melt, fold in the walnuts, and adjust the taste with salt.
9. Spoon the cauliflower grits into serving bowls and top with the stewed tofu.

Nutrition:

Calories: 651, Total Fat: 53.9g, Saturated Fat:23.6 g, Total Carbs: 19 g, Dietary Fiber:5 g, Sugar: 6g, Protein: 32g, Sodium:423 mg

Tempeh Mushroom Omelet

Preparation Time: 10 minutes

Cooking Time: 20 minutes

Serving: 2

Ingredients:

- 2 tbsp olive oil
- 2 oz tempeh, crumbled
- 1 small white onion, chopped
- Salt and black pepper to taste
- 2 tbsp butter
- 6 eggs
- ¼ cup sliced cremini mushrooms
- 2 oz shredded cheddar cheese

Directions:

1. Heat half of the olive oil in a medium frying pan, add the tempeh, season with salt and black pepper, and fry until brown, 10 minutes. Transfer to a plate and set aside.

2. Heat the remaining olive oil in the pan and sauté the onion and mushrooms until softened, 8 minutes. Spoon to the side of the tempeh and set aside.
3. Melt the butter in the pan over low heat.
4. Beat the eggs with some salt, black pepper, and pour into the pan. Swirl to spread the egg around the pan and once the omelet begins to firm, top with the tempeh, mushroom-onion mixture, and cheddar cheese.
5. Use a spatula to carefully release the egg from around the edges of the pan and flip the egg over the stuffing.
6. Once beneath the eggs start to golden brown, 2 minutes, slide the eggs onto a serving plate.
7. Using a knife, divide into half and serve warm.

Nutrition:

Calories:355, Total Fat:29.9 g, Saturated Fat:12.5 g, Total Carbs: 4 g, Dietary Fiber:0 g, Sugar: g, Protein: 18g, Sodium: 324mg

Tempeh Coconut Curry Bake

Preparation Time: 7 minutes

Cooking Time: 23 minutes

Serving: 4

Ingredients:

- 1 oz. plant butter, for greasing
- 2 ½ cups chopped tempeh
- 4 tbsp plant butter
- 2 tbsp red curry paste
- 1 ½ cup coconut cream
- Salt and black pepper
- ½ cup fresh parsley, chopped
- 15 oz. cauliflower, cut into florets

Directions:

1. Preheat the oven to 400 °F and grease a baking dish with 1 ounce of butter.
2. Arrange the tempeh in the baking dish, sprinkle with salt and black pepper, and top each tempeh with a slice of the remaining butter.

3. In a bowl, mix the red curry paste with the coconut cream and parsley. Pour the mixture over the tempeh.
4. Bake in the oven for 20 minutes or until the tempeh is cooked.
5. While baking, season the cauliflower with salt, place in a microwave-safe bowl, and sprinkle with some water. Steam in the microwave for 3 minutes or until the cauliflower is soft and tender within.
6. Remove the curry bake and serve with the caulis.

Nutrition:

Calories:417, Total Fat:38.8g, Saturated Fat:22.4g, Total Carbs: 11g, Dietary Fiber:2g, Sugar: 3g, Protein: 11g, Sodium: 194mg

Tempeh Garam Masala Bake

Preparation Time: 5minutes

Cooking Time: 24minutes

Serving: 4

Ingredients:

- 3 tbsp butter
- 3 cups tempeh slices
- 2 tbsp garam masala
- 1 green bell pepper, finely diced
- Salt
- 1¼ cups coconut cream
- 1 tbsp fresh cilantro, finely chopped

Directions:

1. Preheat the oven to 400 F.
2. Place a skillet over medium heat, add, and melt the butter. Meanwhile, season the tempeh with some salt.
3. Fry the tempeh in the butter until browned on both sides, about 4 minutes.

4. Stir half of the garam masala into the tempeh until evenly mixed; turn the heat off.
5. Transfer the tempeh with the spice into a baking dish.
6. Then, in a small bowl, mix the green bell pepper, coconut cream, cilantro, and remaining garam masala.
7. Pour the mixture over the tempeh and bake in the oven for 20 minutes or until golden brown on top.
8. Garnish with cilantro and serve with some cauli rice.

Nutrition:

Calories:286, Total Fat:27g, Saturated Fat:15g, Total Carbs: 5g, Dietary Fiber:0g, Sugar:1g, Protein:9g, Sodium:87mg

Jalapeno Zucchinis Mix

Preparation time: 10 minutes

Cooking time: 30 minutes

Servings: 4

Ingredients:

- 1 pound zucchinis, sliced
- ¼ cup green onions, chopped
- 1 cup coconut cream
- ½ cup cashew cheese, shredded
- 2 jalapenos, chopped
- Salt and black pepper to the taste
- 2 tablespoons chives, chopped

Directions:

1. In a baking dish, combine the zucchinis with the onions and the other ingredients, toss, bake at 390 degrees F for 30 minutes, divide between plates and serve.

Nutrition:

calories 120, fat 4.2, fiber 2.3, carbs 3, protein 6

Creamy Eggplant Mix

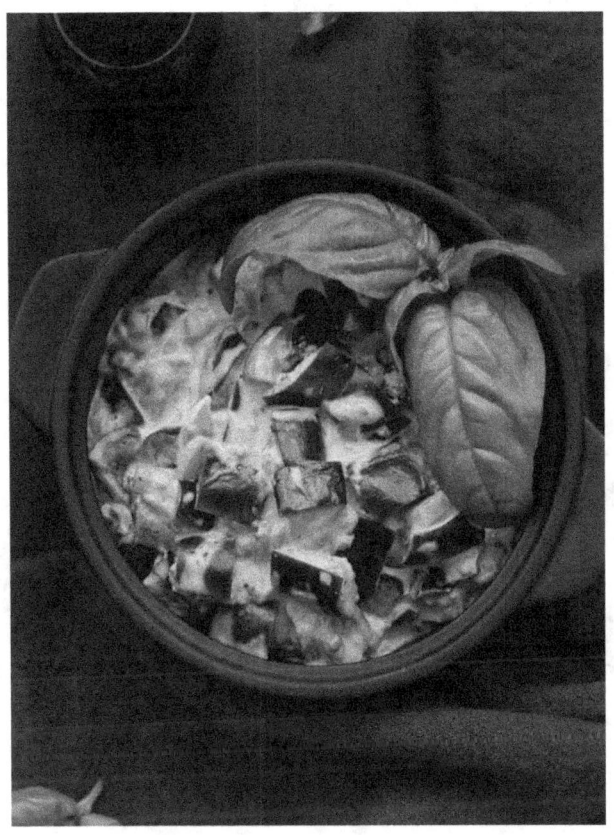

Preparation time: 10 minutes

Cooking time: 15 minutes

Servings: 4

Ingredients:

- 1 pound eggplants, roughly cubed
- 2 scallions, chopped
- ½ cup coconut cream
- 2 tablespoon avocado oil
- 2 teaspoons garlic, minced
- 2 teaspoons chili paste

Directions:

1. Heat up a pan with the oil over medium heat, add the scallions and the garlic and sauté for 2 minutes.
2. Add the eggplants and the other ingredients, toss, cook over medium heat for 13 minutes more, divide between plates and serve as a side dish.

Nutrition:

calories 142, fat 7, fiber 4, carbs 5, protein 3

Chives Kale and Tomato

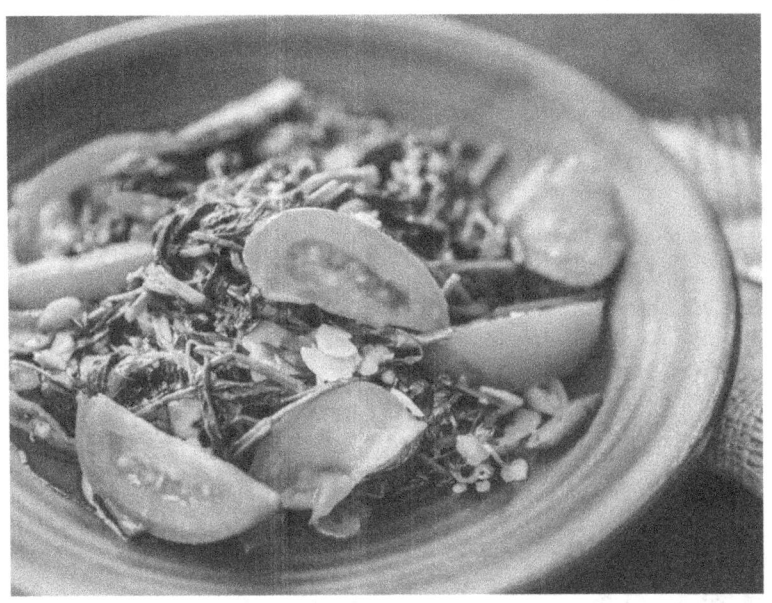

Preparation time: 10 minutes

Cooking time: 20 minutes

Servings: 4

Ingredients:

- 1 pound kale, torn
- ½ pound tomatoes, cut into wedges
- 1 teaspoon chili powder
- 2 tablespoons avocado oil

- 1 teaspoon garam masala
- Salt and black pepper to the taste
- ¼ teaspoon coriander, ground
- A pinch of cayenne pepper
- 1 teaspoon mustard powder
- ¼ cup chives, chopped

Directions:

1. In a roasting pan, combine the kale with the tomatoes and the other ingredients, toss and bake at 380 degrees F for 20 minutes.
2. Divide the mix between plates and serve as a side dish.

Nutrition:

calories 128, fat 2.3, fiber 1, carbs 3.3, protein 4

Ginger Mushrooms

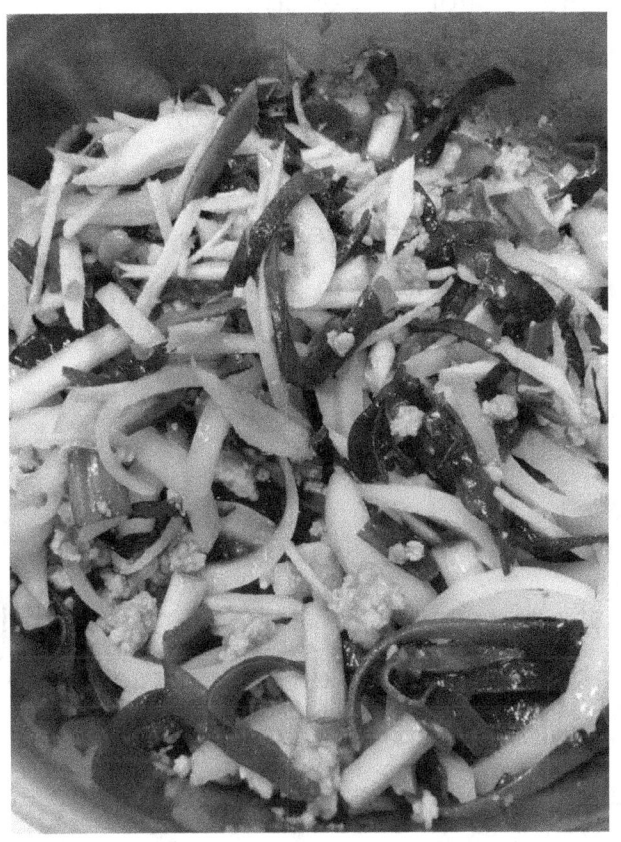

Preparation time: 10 minutes

Cooking time: 20 minutes

Servings: 4

Ingredients:

- 1 pound mushrooms, sliced
- 1 yellow onion, chopped
- 1 tablespoon ginger, grated
- 2 tablespoons balsamic vinegar
- 1 tablespoon olive oil
- 2 garlic cloves, minced
- A pinch of salt and black pepper
- ¼ cup lime juice
- 2 tablespoons walnuts, chopped

Directions:

1. Heat up a pan with the oil over medium-high heat, add the onion and the ginger and sauté for 5 minutes.
2. Add the mushrooms and the other ingredients, toss, cook over medium heat for 15 minutes more, divide between plates and serve.

Nutrition:

calories 120, fat 2, fiber 2, carbs 4, protein 5

Basil Green Beans

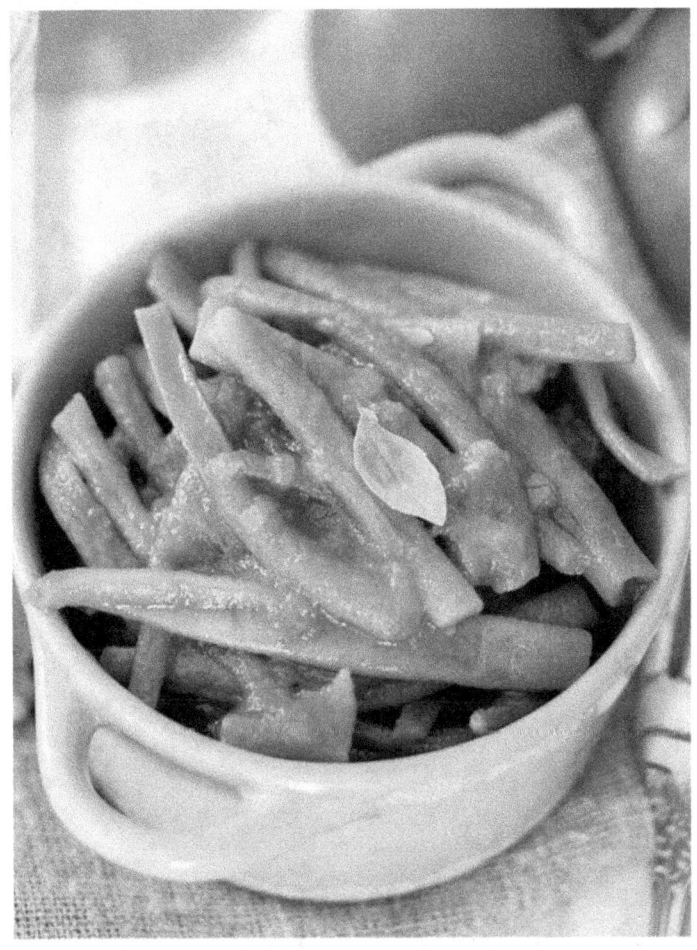

Preparation time: 10 minutes

Cooking time: 20 minutes

Servings: 4

Ingredients:

- 1 yellow onion, chopped
- 1 pound green beans, trimmed and halved
- 1 tablespoon tomato sauce
- 1 tablespoon avocado oil
- 2 teaspoons basil, dried
- A pinch of salt and black pepper

Directions:

1. Heat up a pan with the oil over medium-high heat, add the onion and sauté for 5 minutes.
2. Add the green beans and the other ingredients, toss, cook for 15 minutes more.
3. Divide everything between plates and serve as a side dish.

Nutrition:

calories 221, fat 5, fiber 8, carbs 10, protein 8

Cauliflower and Chives Mash

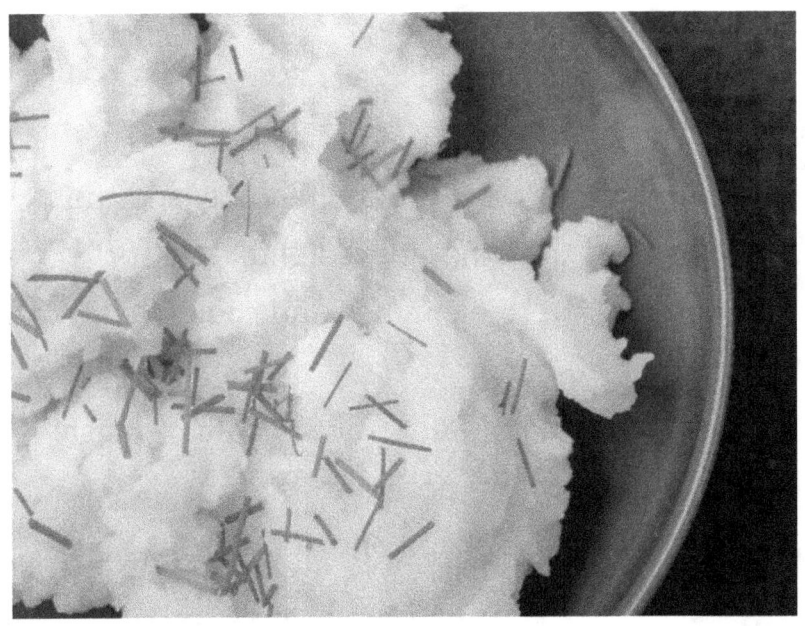

Preparation time: 10 minutes

Cooking time: 20 minutes

Servings: 4

Ingredients:

- 2 pounds cauliflower florets
- 2 cups water
- 1 teaspoon cumin, dried
- 1 teaspoon thyme, dried

- 1 cup coconut cream
- 2 garlic cloves, minced
- A pinch of salt and black pepper

Directions:

1. Put the cauliflower florets in a pot, add the water and the other ingredients except the cream, bring to a simmer and cook over medium heat for 20 minutes.
2. Drain the cauliflower, add the cream, mash everything with a potato masher, whisk well, divide between plates and serve.

Nutrition:

calories 200, fat 14.7, fiber 7.2, carbs 16.3, protein 6.1

Crispy Zucchini Fries

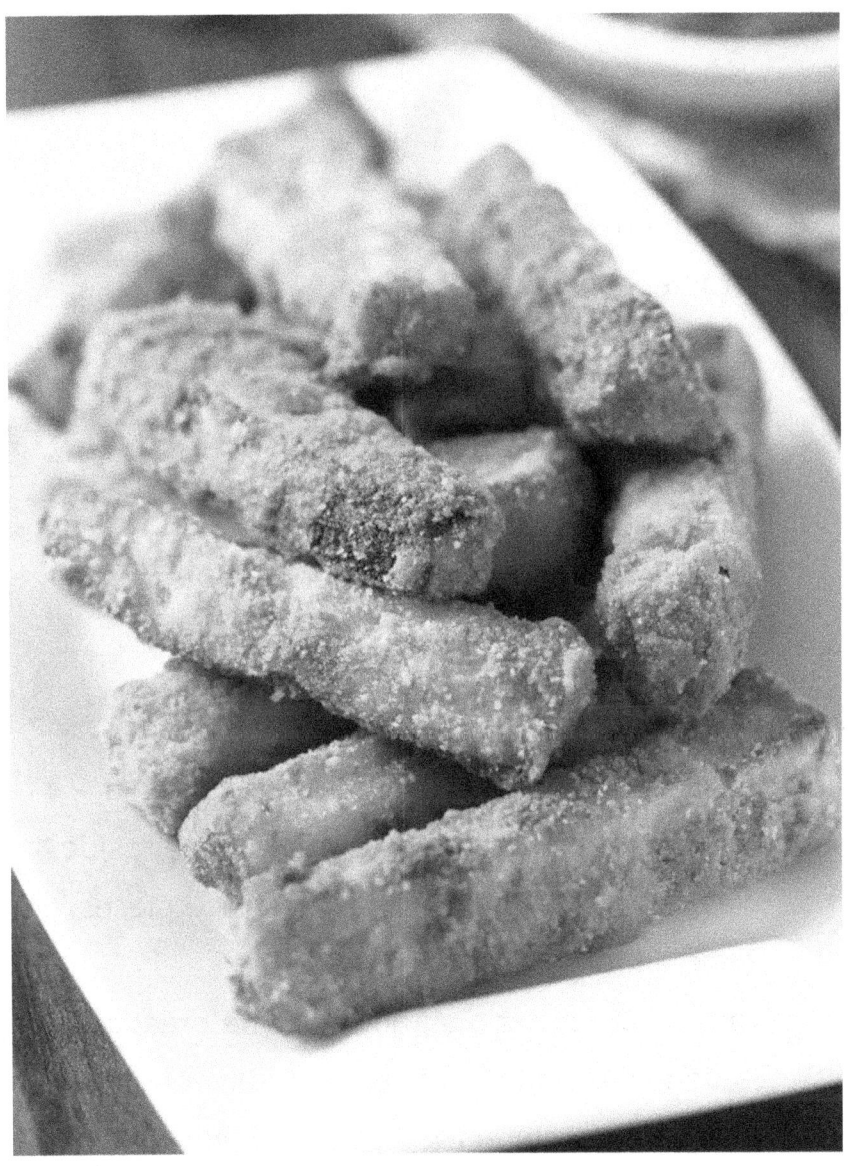

Preparation Time: 10 minutes

Cooking Time: 25 minutes

Servings: 4

Ingredients:

- 1 medium zucchini
- 4 tablespoons almond meal
- 4 tablespoons light ranch dressing
- 2 teaspoons Italian seasoning
- 3 tablespoons Franks hot sauce
- ½ cup breadcrumbs
- 2 tablespoons Parmesan cheese, grated

Directions:

1. Preheat oven to 395° Fahrenheit. Spray a baking dish with cooking spray and set aside.
2. Wash zucchini and cut into fries' size pieces. Place almond meal in a flat dish.
3. Take another flat dish and mix the breadcrumbs, Italian seasoning, and cheese on it.
4. In a bowl combine the hot sauce and ranch dressing.

5. Roll zucchini pieces in the almond meal then dip in sauce mixture and finally coat with breadcrumb mixture.
6. Place coated zucchini on prepared baking dish.
7. Bake in preheated oven for 25 minutes.
8. Flip zucchini fries once halfway through.
9. Serve and enjoy!

Nutrition:

Calories: 149 Sugar: 2.6 g Cholesterol: 11 mg Fat: 8.1 g Carbohydrates: 13.6 g Proteins: 6 g

Cajun Sweet Potatoes

Preparation time: 5 minutes

cooking time: 30 minutes

servings: 4

Ingredients

- 2 pounds sweet potatoes
- 2 teaspoons extra-virgin olive oil
- ½ teaspoon ground cayenne pepper
- ½ teaspoon dried oregano
- ½ teaspoon dried thyme
- ½ teaspoon smoked paprika
- ½ teaspoon garlic powder
- ½ teaspoon salt (optional)

Directions

1. Preheat the oven to 400 °F. Line a baking sheet with parchment paper.
2. Wash the potatoes, pat dry, and cut into ¾-inch cubes. Transfer to a large bowl, and pour the olive oil over the potatoes.

3. In a small bowl, combine the cayenne, paprika, oregano, thyme, and garlic powder.
4. Sprinkle the spices over the potatoes and combine until the potatoes are well coated.
5. Spread the potatoes on the prepared baking sheet in a single layer.
6. Season with the salt (if using).
7. Roast for 30 minutes, stirring the potatoes after 15 minutes.
8. Divide the potatoes evenly among 4 single-serving containers. Let cool completely before sealing.

Nutrition:

Calories: 219; Fat: 3g; Protein: 4g; Carbohydrates: 46g; Fiber: 7g; Sugar: 9g; Sodium: 125mg

Miso Spaghetti Squash

Preparation time: 5 minutes

cooking time: 40 minutes

servings: 4

Ingredients

- 1 (3-poundspaghetti squash
- 1 tablespoon hot water
- 1 tablespoon unseasoned rice vinegar
- 1 tablespoon white miso

Directions

1. Preheat the oven to 400 °F.
2. Line a rimmed baking sheet with parchment paper.
3. Halve the squash lengthwise and place, cut-side down, on the prepared baking sheet.
4. Bake for 35 to 40 minutes, until tender.
5. Cool until the squash is easy to handle.
6. With a fork, scrape out the flesh, which will be stringy, like spaghetti.

7. Transfer to a large bowl.
8. In a small bowl, combine the hot water, vinegar, and miso with a whisk or fork.
9. Pour over the squash. Gently toss with tongs to coat the squash.
10. Divide the squash evenly among 4 single-serving containers.
11. Let cool before sealing the lids.

Nutrition:

Calories: 117; Fat: 2g; Protein: 3g; Carbohydrates: 25g; Fiber: 0g; Sugar: 0g; Sodium: 218mg

Baked Potatoes and "BBQ" Lentils

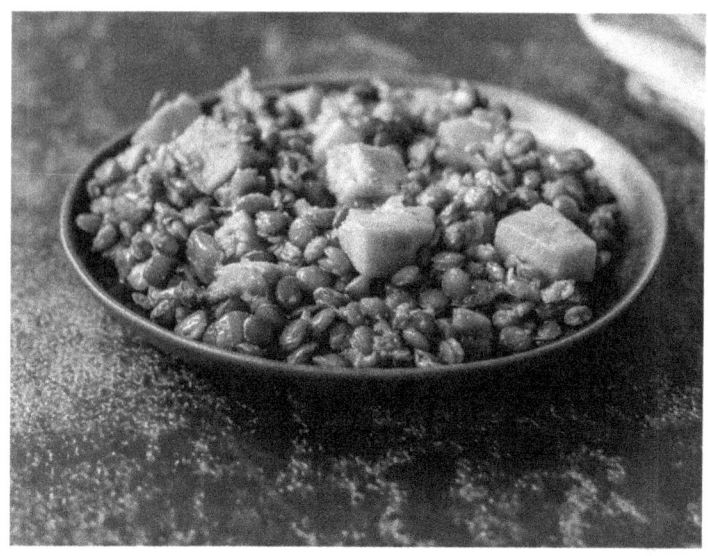

Preparation Time: 5 mins

Servings: 4

Ingredients:

- 2 sliced large baked potatoes
- 1 c. dry brown lentils
- 1 chopped small onion
- 2 tsps. molasses
- 2 tsps. liquid smoke
- 3 c. water

- ½ c. organic ketchup

Directions:

1. Add water, onion and lentils to the pot
2. Lock up the lid and cook on HIGH pressure for 10 minutes
3. Release the pressure naturally
4. Add ketchup, liquid smoke and molasses to the lentil
5. Sauté for 5 minutes
6. Serve over baked potatoes and enjoy!

Nutrition:

Calories: 140, Fat:4 g, Carbs:24 g, Protein:5 g, Sugars:606 g, Sodium:18 mg

Fresh Fruit Smoothie

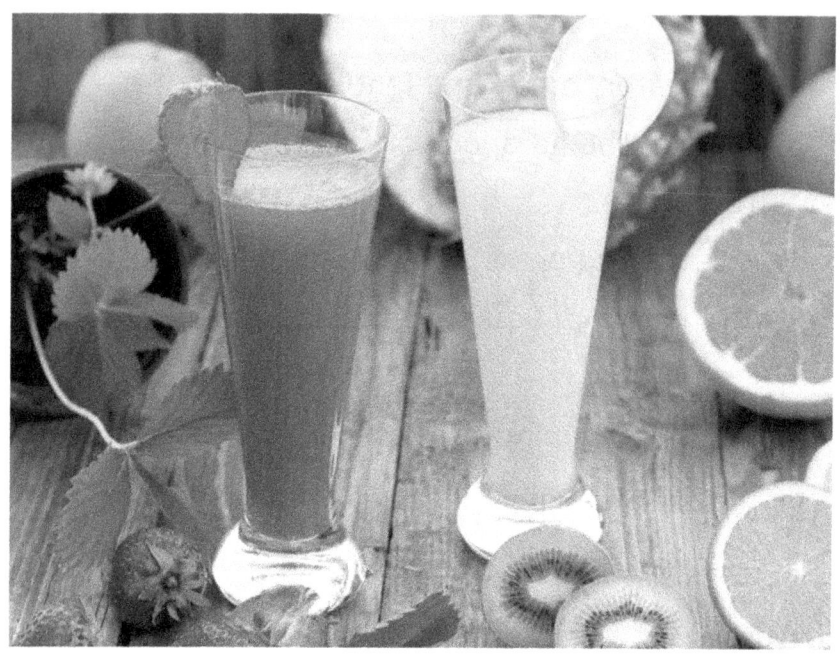

Preparation Time: 5 mins

Servings: 4

Ingredients:

- 1 tbsp. honey
- 1 c. fresh strawberries
- 1 c. fresh pineapple
- 2 orange juice

- ½ c. cantaloupe
- 1 c. water

Directions:

1. Remove the rind from the melon and pineapple. Cut them into chunks and remove the stems from the strawberries.
2. Put everything in a blender and serve.

Nutrition:

Calories: 72, Fat:1 g, Carbs:17 g, Protein:1 g, Sugars:1 g, Sodium:42 mg

Green Vegetable Smoothie

Preparation Time: 5 mins

Servings: 4

Ingredients:

- 1 c. cold water
- ½ c. strawberries
- 2 oz. baby spinach
- 1 lemon juice
- 1 tbsp. fresh mint
- 1 banana
- ½ c. blueberries

Directions:

1. Put all the ingredients in a juicer or blender and puree.

Nutrition:

Calories: 52, Fat:2 g, Carbs:12 g, Protein:1 g, Sugars:18 g, Sodium:36 mg

Celery Stew

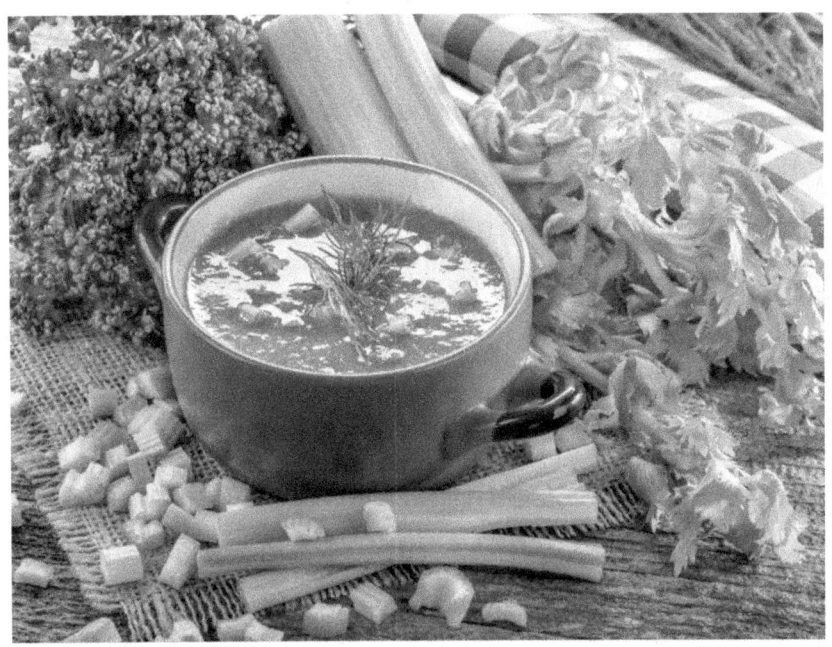

Preparation time: 10 minutes

Cooking time: 30 minutes

Servings: 6

Ingredients:

- 1 celery bunch, chopped
- 1 bunch green onion, peeled and chopped
- 1 onion, peeled and chopped

- 4 garlic cloves, peeled and minced
- Salt and ground black pepper, to taste
- 1 fresh parsley bunch, chopped
- 2 fresh mint bunches, chopped
- 3 dried Persian lemons, pricked with a fork
- 2 cups water
- 2 teaspoons chicken bouillon
- 4 tablespoons olive oil

Directions:

1. Heat up a pot with the oil over medium-high heat, add the onion, green onions, and garlic, stir, and cook for 6 minutes.
2. Add the celery, Persian lemons, chicken bouillon, salt, pepper, and water, stir, cover pot, and simmer on medium heat for 20 minutes.
3. Add the parsley and mint, stir, and cook for 10 minutes.
4. Divide into bowls and serve.

Nutrition:

Calories - 170, Fat - 7, Fiber - 4, Carbs - 6, Protein - 10

Sautéed Mustard Greens

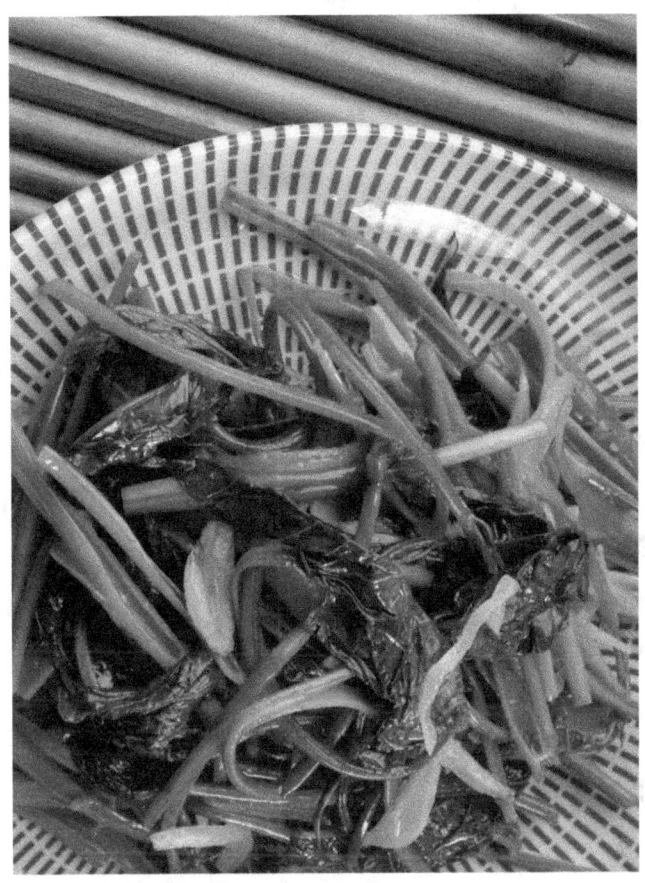

Preparation time: 5 minutes

Cooking time: 15 minutes

Servings: 4

Ingredients:

- 1 pound mustard greens, torn
- 2 garlic cloves, peeled and minced
- 1 tablespoon olive oil
- ½ cup onion, sliced
- Salt and ground black pepper, to taste
- 3 tablespoons vegetable stock
- ¼ teaspoon dark sesame oil

Directions:

1. Heat up a pan with the oil over medium heat, add the onions, stir, and brown them for 10 minutes.
2. Add the garlic, stir, and cook for 1 minute.
3. Add the stock, greens, salt, and pepper, stir, and cook for 5 minutes.
4. Add more salt and pepper, and sesame oil, toss to coat, divide on plates, and serve.

Nutrition:

Calories - 120, Fat - 3, Fiber - 1, Carbs - 3, Protein - 6

Roasted Asparagus

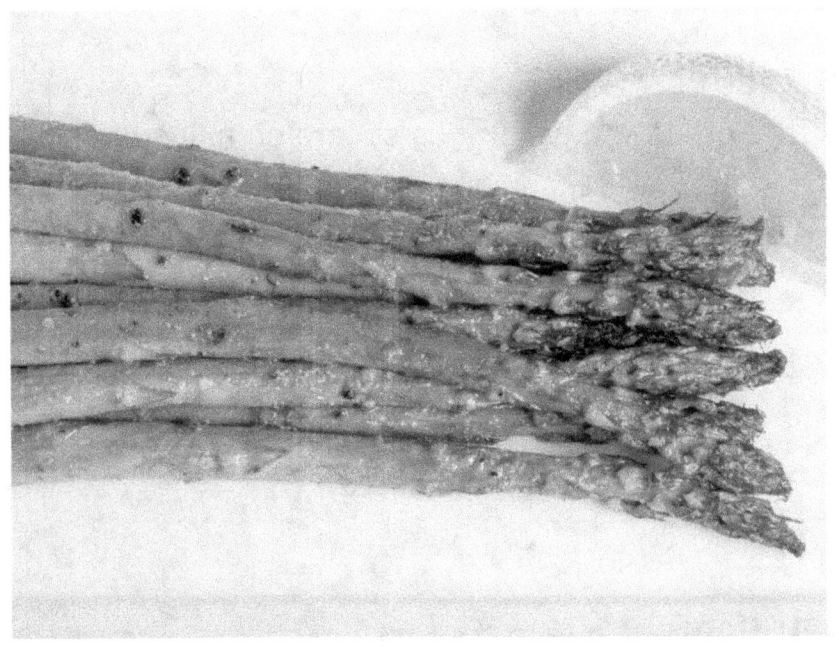

Preparation time: 10 minutes

Cooking time: 10 minutes

Servings: 3

Ingredients:

- 1 asparagus bunch, trimmed
- 3 teaspoons avocado oil
- A splash of lemon juice

- 1 tablespoon fresh oregano, chopped
- Salt and ground black pepper, to taste

Directions:

1. Spread the asparagus spears on a lined baking sheet, season with salt, and pepper, drizzle with oil and lemon juice, sprinkle with oregano, and toss to coat well.
2. Place in an oven at 425 °F, and bake for 10 minutes.
3. Divide on plates and serve.

Nutrition:

Calories - 130, Fat - 1, Fiber - 1, Carbs - 2, Protein - 3

Arugula and Broccoli Soup

Preparation time: 10 minutes

Cooking time: 20 minutes

Servings: 4

Ingredients:

- 1 broccoli head, separated into florets
- 1 onion, peeled and chopped
- 1 tablespoon olive oil
- 1 garlic clove, peeled and minced
- Salt and ground black pepper, to taste
- 2, and ½ cups vegetable stock
- 1 teaspoon cumin
- Juice of ½ lemon
- 1 cup arugula leaves

Directions:

1. Heat up a pot with the oil over medium-high heat, add the onions, stir, and cook for 4 minutes.
2. Add the garlic, stir, and cook for 1 minute.

3. Add the broccoli, cumin, salt, and pepper, stir, and cook for 4 minutes.
4. Add the stock, stir, and cook for 8 minutes.
5. Blend the soup using an immersion blender, add half of the arugula, and blend again.
6. Add the rest of the arugula, stir, and heat up the soup again.
7. Add the lemon juice, stir, ladle into soup bowls, and serve.

Nutrition:

Calories - 150, Fat - 3, Fiber - 1, Carbs - 3, Protein - 7

Basil Tomato Soup

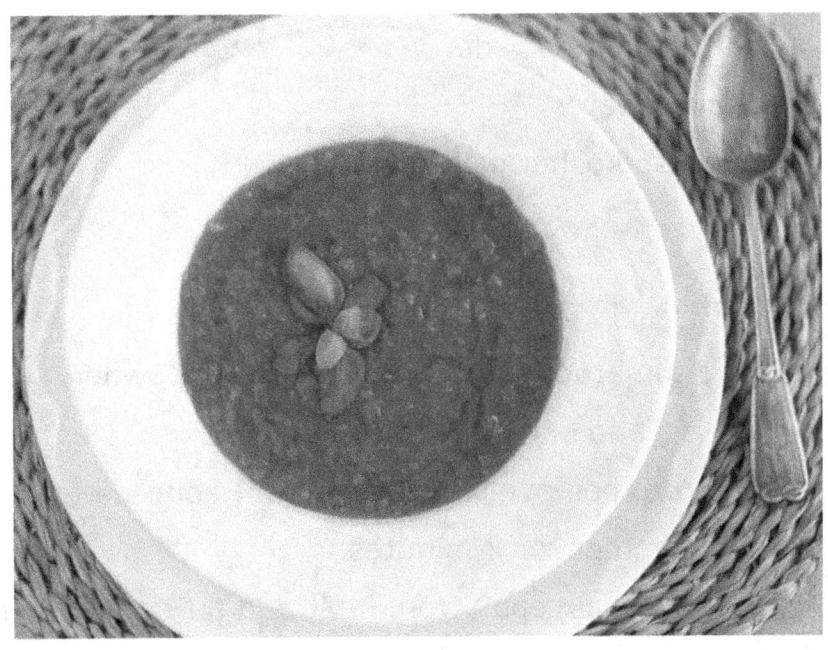

Preparation Time: 5 minutes

Cooking Time: 15 minutes

Servings: 6

Ingredients:

- 28 oz can tomatoes
- ¼ tsp dried basil leaves
- ¼ cup basil pesto

- 1 tsp apple cider vinegar
- 2 tbsp erythritol
- ¼ tsp garlic powder
- ½ tsp onion powder
- 2 cups water
- 1 ½ tsp kosher salt

Directions:

1. Add tomatoes, garlic powder, onion powder, water, and salt in a saucepan.
2. Bring to boil over medium heat. Reduce heat and simmer for 2 minutes.
3. Remove saucepan from heat and puree the soup using a blender until smooth.
4. Stir in pesto, dried basil, vinegar, and erythritol.
5. Stir well and serve warm.

Nutrition:

Calories 30, Fat 0g, Carbohydrates 12.1g, Sugar 9.6g, Protein 1.3g, Cholesterol 0mg

Black Bean Soup With A Splash

Preparation Time: 5 Minutes

Cooking Time: 45 Minutes

Servings: 4 To 6

Ingredients

- 1 tablespoon olive oil
- 1 medium onion, finely chopped
- 1 celery rib, finely chopped
- 2 medium carrots, finely chopped
- 1 small green bell pepper, finely chopped
- 2 garlic cloves, minced
- 4 1/2 cups cooked or 3 (15.5-ounce) cans black beans, drained and rinsed
- 4 cups vegetable broth, homemade (see Light Vegetable Broth) or store-bought, or water
- 1 teaspoon dried thyme
- 1 teaspoon salt
- 1/4 teaspoon ground cayenne
- 2 tablespoons minced fresh parsley, for garnish
- 1/3 cup dry sherry

Directions

1. In a large soup pot, heat the oil over medium heat. Add the onion, celery, carrots, bell pepper, and garlic. Cover and cook until tender, stirring occasionally, about 10 minutes.
2. Add the broth, beans, thyme, salt, and cayenne. Bring to a boil, then reduce the heat to low and simmer, uncovered, until the soup has thickened, about 45 minutes.
3. Puree the soup in the pot with an immersion blender or in a blender or food processor, in batches if necessary, and return to the pot. Reheat if necessary.
4. Ladle the soup into bowls and garnish with parsley. Serve accompanied by the sherry.

Coconut Tofu Zucchini Bake

Preparation Time: 40 minutes

Serving: 4

Ingredients:

- 1 tbsp butter
- 1 cup green beans, chopped
- 1 bunch asparagus, trimmed and cut into 1-inch pieces
- 2 cups coconut milk
- 2 tbsp arrowroot starch
- 4 medium zucchinis, spiralized
- 1 cup grated parmesan cheese
- 1 (15 oz) firm tofu, pressed and sliced
- Salt and black pepper to taste

Directions:

1. Preheat the oven to 380 °F.
2. Melt the butter in a medium skillet and sauté the green beans and asparagus until softened, about 5 minutes. Set aside.

3. In a medium saucepan, mix the arrowroot starch with the coconut milk. Bring to a boil over medium heat with frequent stirring until thickened, 3 minutes. Stir in half of the parmesan cheese until melted.
4. Mix in the green beans, asparagus, zucchinis and tofu. Season with salt and black pepper.
5. Transfer the mixture to a baking dish and cover the top with the remaining parmesan cheese.
6. Bake in the oven until the cheese melts and golden on top, 20 minutes.
7. Remove the food from the oven and serve warm.

Nutrition:

Calories: 492, Total Fat:26.8 g, Saturated Fat: 12.6g, Total Carbs: 14g, Dietary Fiber:4g, Sugar: 8g, Protein: 50g, Sodium: 1668mg

Creamy Avocado-Dressed Kale Salad

Preparation time: 10 minutes

cooking time: 20 minutes

servings: 4

Ingredients

For The Dressing

- 1 avocado, peeled and pitted
- 1 tablespoon fresh lemon juice, or 1 teaspoon lemon juice concentrate and 2 teaspoons water
- 1 scallion, chopped
- 1 tablespoon fresh or dried dill1 small garlic clove, pressed
- Pinch sea salt
- ¼ cup water

For The Salad

- 8 large kale leaves
- 1 cup cherry tomatoes, halved
- ½ cup chopped green beans, raw or lightly steamed
- 1 bell pepper, chopped
- 2 scallions, chopped

- 2 cups cooked millet, or other cooked whole grain, such as quinoa or brown rice
- Hummus (optional)

Directions

To Make The Dressing

1. Put all the ingredients in a blender or food processor.
2. Purée until smooth, then add water as necessary to get the consistency you're looking for in your dressing.
3. Taste for seasoning, and add more salt if you need to.

To Make The Salad

4. Chop the kale, removing the stems if you want your salad less bitter, and then massage the leaves with your fingers until it wilts and gets a bit moist, about 2 minutes.
5. You can use a pinch salt if you like to help it soften.
6. Toss the kale with the green beans, cherry tomatoes, bell pepper, scallions, millet, and the dressing.

7. Pile the salad onto plates, and top them off with a spoonful of hummus (if using).

Nutrition

Calories: 225; Total fat: 7g; Carbs: 37g; Fiber: 7g; Protein: 7g

Classic Potato Salad

Preparation Time: 10 Minutes

Cooking Time: 15 Minutes

Servings: 4

Ingredients

- 6 potatoes, scrubbed or peeled and chopped
- Pinch salt
- 4 celery stalks, chopped
- ½ cup Creamy Tahini Dressing or vegan mayo
- 1 teaspoon dried dill (optional)
- 1 teaspoon Dijon mustard (optional)
- 2 scallions, white and light green parts only, chopped

Directions

1. Put the potatoes in a large pot, add the salt, and pour in enough water to cover. Bring the water to a boil over high heat.
2. Cook the potatoes for 15 to 20 minutes, until soft.

3. Drain and set aside to cool. (Alternatively, put the potatoes in a large microwave-safe dish with a bit of water. Cover and heat on high power for 10 minutes.)
4. In a large bowl, whisk together the dressing, dill (if using), and mustard (if using).
5. Toss the celery and scallions with the dressing.
6. Add the cooked, cooled potatoes and toss to combine.
7. Store leftovers in an airtight container in the refrigerator for up to 1 week.

Nutrition Per Serving

Calories: 269; Protein: 6g; Total fat: 5g; Saturated fat: 1g; Carbohydrates: 51g; Fiber: 6g

Garden Salad Wraps

Preparation time: 15 minutes

cooking time: 10 minutes

servings: 4 wraps

Ingredients

- 6 tablespoons olive oil
- 1 pound extra-firm tofu, drained, patted dry, and cut into 1/2-inch strips
- 1/4 cup apple cider vinegar
- 1 tablespoon soy sauce
- 1 teaspoon yellow or spicy brown mustard
- 1/2 teaspoon salt
- 1/4 teaspoon freshly ground black pepper
- 3 ripe Roma tomatoes, finely chopped
- 3 cups shredded romaine lettuce
- 1 large carrot, shredded
- 1 medium English cucumber, peeled and chopped
- 1/3 cup minced red onion
- 1/4 cup sliced pitted green olives
- 4 (10-inchwhole-grain flour tortillas or lavash flatbread

Directions

1. In a large skillet, heat 2 tablespoons of the oil over medium heat. Add the tofu and cook until golden brown, about 10 minutes. Sprinkle with soy sauce and set aside to cool.
2. In a small bowl, combine the vinegar, mustard, salt, and pepper with the remaining 4 tablespoons oil, stirring to blend well. Set aside.
3. In a large bowl, combine the lettuce, tomatoes, carrot, cucumber, onion, and olives. Pour on the dressing and toss to coat.
4. To assemble wraps, place 1 tortilla on a work surface and spread with about one-quarter of the salad. Place a few strips of tofu on the tortilla and roll up tightly. Slice in half

Almond Lemon Biscuits

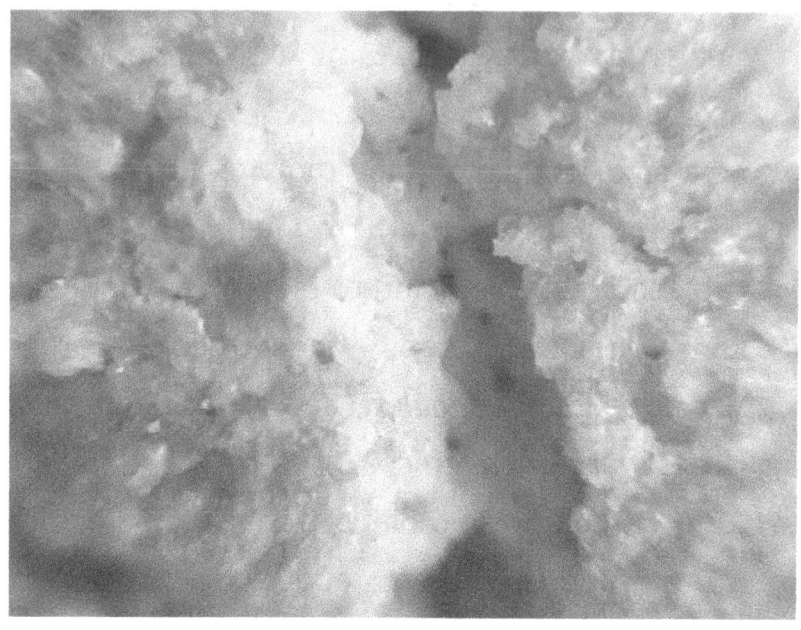

Preparation Time: 10 minutes

Cooking Time: 12-15 minutes

Servings: 6

Ingredients:

- 3 c. almond flour
- ½ c. unsalted grass-fed butter
- 2 eggs
- 3 tbsps. Stevia

- 1 tbsp. fresh lemon juice
- 1½ tsps. Baking powder

Directions:

1. Preheat oven to 350 ºF.
2. Combine the almond flour, Stevia and baking powder in a bowl.
3. Whisk the eggs in a separate bowl.
4. Melt the butter, and combine with almond flour, lemon juice and eggs mixture; stir well.
5. Divide the mixture equally into 6 biscuits and place in a greased baking dish.
6. Bake for 12-15 minutes.
7. Let cool on a wire rack.
8. Serve warm or cold.

Nutrition:

Calories: 27, Fat: 25.91g, Carbs: 4.49g, Protein 5.9g

Zesty Orange-Cranberry Energy Bites

Preparation Time: 10 minutes

Chill Time: 15 minutes

Serves: 12 bites

Ingredients:

- 2 tablespoons almond butter, or cashew or sunflower seed butter
- 1 tablespoon chia seeds
- 2 tablespoons maple syrup, or brown rice syrup
- ¾ cup cooked quinoa
- ¼ cup sesame seeds, toasted
- ½ teaspoon almond extract, or vanilla extract
- Zest of 1 orange
- 1 tablespoon dried cranberries
- ¼ cup ground almonds

Directions:

1. In a medium bowl, mix together the nut or seed butter and syrup until smooth and creamy.
2. Stir in the rest of the ingredients, and mix to make sure the consistency is holding together in

a ball. Form the mix into 12 balls.
3. Place them on a baking sheet lined with parchment or waxed paper and put in the fridge to set for about 15 minutes.
4. If your balls aren't holding together, it's likely because of the moisture content of your cooked quinoa.
5. Add more nut or seed butter mixed with syrup until it all sticks together.

Nutrition (1 bite):

Calories: 109; total fat: 7g, Carbs: 11g, Fiber: 3g, Protein: 3g

Pumpkin Spice Cake.

Preparation Time: 28 Minutes

Servings: 6

Ingredients:

- 1¾ cups unbleached all-purpose flour
- 1 cup canned solid-pack pumpkin
- ½ cup chopped pecans
- ¾ cup packed light brown sugar or granulated natural sugar
- ¼ cup unsweetened almond milk
- ¼ cup vegetable oil
- 1½ teaspoons baking powder
- 1 teaspoon ground cinnamon
- 1 teaspoon pure vanilla extract
- ½ teaspoon salt
- ½ teaspoon ground nutmeg
- ½ teaspoon ground allspice
- ¼ teaspoon ground cloves

Directions:

1. Lightly oil a baking tray that will fit in the steamer basket of your Cooker.
2. In a bowl combine the flour, baking powder, cinnamon, nutmeg, allspice, cloves, sugar, and salt.
3. In another bowl combine the pumpkin, oil, almond milk, and vanilla.
4. Mix the wet and dry mixtures together until the mix is evenly smooth.
5. Fold in the pecans.
6. Pour the batter into your baking tray and put the tray in your steamer basket.
7. Pour the minimum amount of water into the base of your Cooker and lower the steamer basket.
8. Seal and cook on Steam for 12 minutes.
9. Release the pressure quickly and set to one side to cool a little.

Peanut Butter & Chocolate Cheesecake

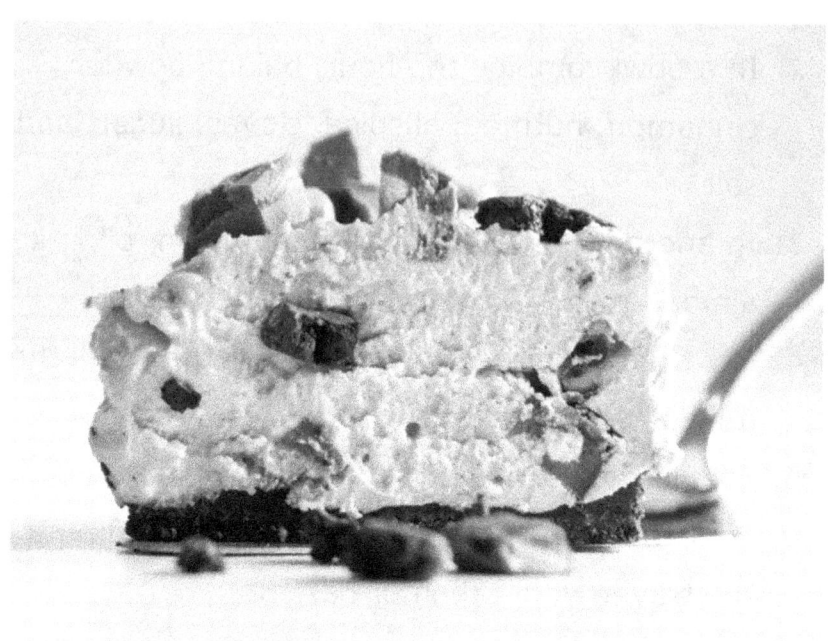

Preparation Time: 30 Minutes

Servings: 8

Ingredients:

- 16 ounces vegan cream cheese
- 8 ounces silken tofu, drained
- ¾ cup natural sugar
- 1½ cups crushed vegan chocolate cookies
- ½ cup creamy peanut butter, at room

temperature
- ¼ cup unsweetened cocoa powder
- 3 tablespoons vegan butter, melted
- 2 tablespoons hazelnut milk

Directions:

1. Lightly oil a baking tray that will fit in the steamer basket of your Cooker.
2. Combine the chocolate crumbs and the butter.
3. Press the chocolate base into your tray.
4. Blend the cream cheese and tofu until smooth.
5. Add the peanut butter, cocoa, hazelnut milk, and sugar to the cheese mix and fold in well.
6. Pour the cheese onto your base and put the tray in your steamer basket.
7. Pour the minimum amount of water into the base of your Cooker and lower the steamer basket.
8. Seal and cook on Steam for 15 minutes.
9. Release the pressure quickly and set to one side to cool a little.

Chocolate Bread Pudding.

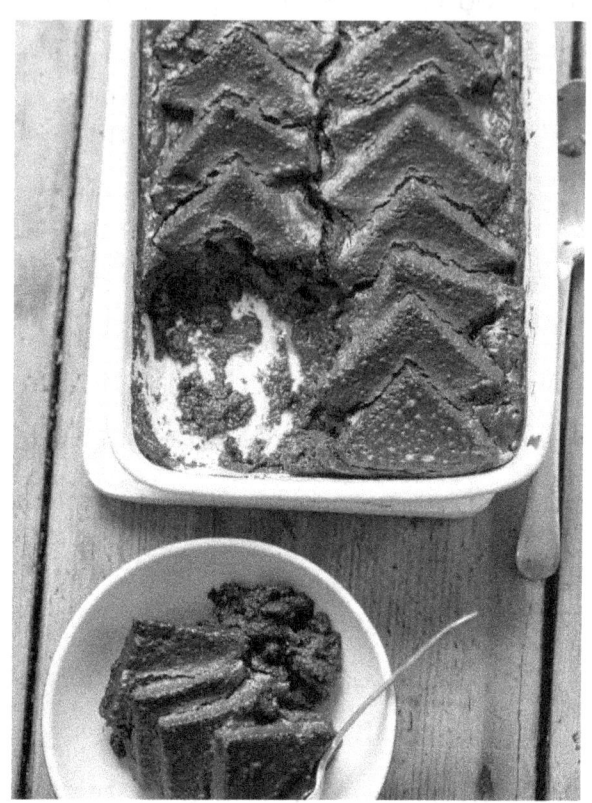

Preparation Time: 40 Minutes

Servings: 6

Ingredients:

- 4 cups white bread cubes
- 2 cups vegan semisweet chocolate chips

- 2 cups unsweetened almond milk
- ½ cup chopped pecans or walnuts
- ¾ cup granulated natural sugar
- ¼ cup unsweetened cocoa powder
- 1 tablespoon vegan butter
- 1 teaspoon pure vanilla extract
- ½ teaspoon salt

Directions:

1. Oil a baking tray that will fit in your Cooker.
2. Melt 1 and 2/3 of the chocolate chips with 1.5 cups of almond milk.
3. Spread the bread cubes in your Cooker, sprinkle with nuts, and the remaining chocolate chips.
4. Warm the remaining almond milk in another saucepan with sugar, cocoa, vanilla, and salt.
5. Combine the cocoa mix with the chocolate chip mix and pour it over the bread.
6. Seal your Cooker and cook on Beans for 30 minutes.
7. Depressurize naturally.

Cheesecake

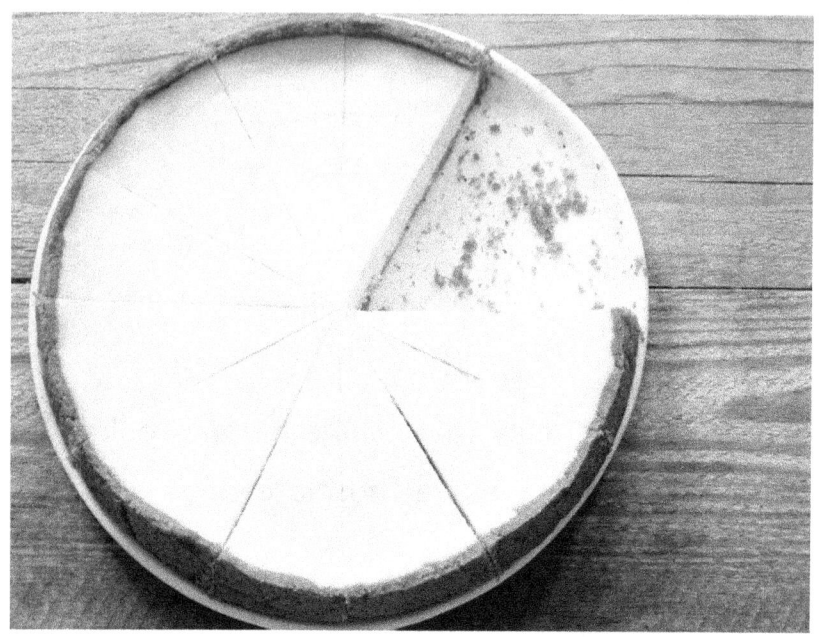

Preparation time: 45 minutes

Ingredients:

For the crust:

- 4 tbsp. butter
- 6 cups coconut, shredded
- 8 Oz. cream cheese
- Any sweetener you consider appropriate
- ½ cup stevia sweetener

- ½ maple syrup
- 16 Oz. can of pineapple in a syrup, crashed or whole, drained
- ¼ cup whipping cream
- 5 eggs

Directions:

1. After you mix all the crust ingredients, press evenly, place it into the baking tray or pan, and have it baked for at least 10 minutes. Let it cool.
2. In a blender mix well the cream cheese with sweeteners, the pineapple until blended.
3. Add the eggs gradually and pour this batter into the pan you have prepared.
4. Bake for 90 minutes. Remove from oven and let it cooled.

Tip: Can be served with additional pineapple on top and/or with whipped cream, whatever topping you choose to your liking.

Berry Cake

Preparation time: 10 minutes

Cooking time: 30 minutes

Servings: 6

Ingredients:

- 2 cups coconut flour
- 1 cup blueberries
- 1 cup strawberries, chopped
- 2 tablespoons almonds, chopped
- 2 tablespoons walnuts, chopped
- 1 teaspoon almond extract
- 3 tablespoons flaxseed mixed with 4 tablespoons water
- ½ cup coconut cream
- 2 tablespoons avocado oil
- 1 teaspoon baking powder
- 3 tablespoons stevia
- Cooking spray

Directions:

1. In a bowl, combine the coconut flour with the berries, the nuts, stevia and the other ingredients, and whisk well.
2. Grease a cake pan with the cooking spray, pour the cake mix inside, introduce everything in the oven at 360 degrees F and bake for 30 minutes.
3. Cool the cake down, slice and serve.

Nutrition:

calories 225, fat 9, fiber 4.5, carbs 10.2, protein 4.5

Cinnamon Avocado and Berries Mix

Preparation time: 5 minutes

Cooking time: 0 minutes

Servings: 4

Ingredients:

- 1 cup blackberries
- 1 cup strawberries, halved
- 1 cup avocado, peeled, pitted and cubed
- 1 teaspoon cinnamon powder
- 1 cup coconut cream
- 4 tablespoons stevia

Directions:

1. In a bowl, combine the berries with the avocado and the other ingredients, toss, divide into smaller bowls and serve cold.

Nutrition:

calories 162, fat 8, fiber 4.2, carbs 12.3, protein 8.4

Chocolate Pudding

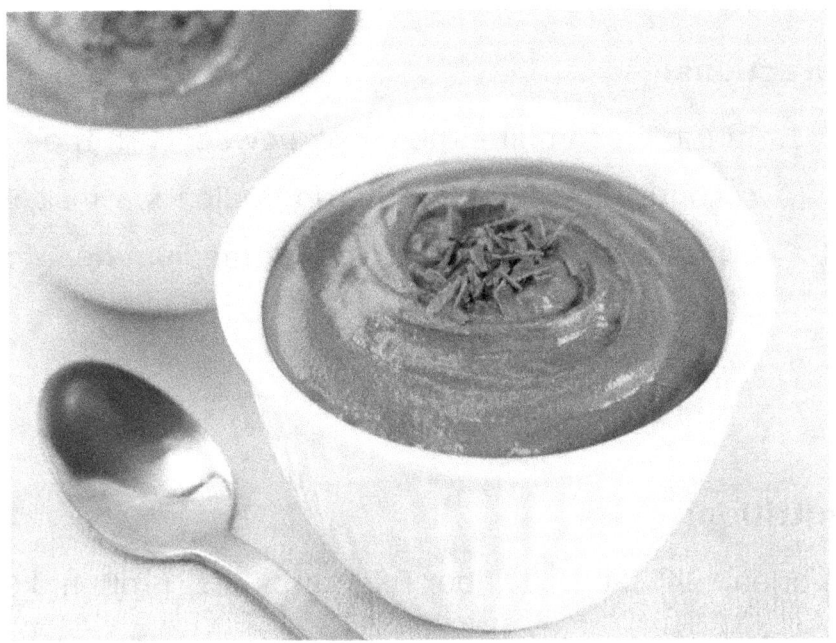

Preparation time: 10 minutes

Cooking time: 20 minutes

Servings: 4

Ingredients:

- 2/3 cup coconut cream
- 2 tablespoons cocoa powder
- 2 tablespoons coconut oil, melted

- 2 tablespoons stevia
- ¼ teaspoon almond extract

Directions:

1. In a pan, combine the cocoa powder with the coconut milk and the other ingredients, whisk, bring to a simmer ad cook over medium heat for 20 minutes.
2. Divide into cups and serve cold.

Nutrition:

calories 134, fat 14.1, fiber 0.8, carbs 3.1, protein 0.9

Grapes Pie

Preparation time: 10 minutes

Cooking time: 40 minutes

Servings: 6

Ingredients:

- ½ cup stevia
- 2 cups grapes, halved
- ½ cup coconut cream
- ½ teaspoon vanilla extract
- 1 cup coconut flour
- 1 teaspoon baking powder
- 3 tablespoons flaxseed mixed with 4 tablespoons water

Directions:

1. In a bowl, combine the grapes with the stevia, vanilla and the other ingredients, whisk well and pour into a pie pan.
2. Bake at 375 degress F for 40 minutes, cool down, slice and serve.

Nutrition:

calories 200, fat 4.4, fiber 3, carbs 7.6, protein 8

Walnuts Cream

Preparation time: 10 minutes

Cooking time: 0 minutes

Servings: 4

Ingredients:

- Juice of 1 lime
- ½ cup stevia
- ½ cup walnuts, chopped
- 3 cups coconut milk
- ½ cup coconut cream
- 2 teaspoons cardamom, ground
- 1 teaspoon vanilla extract

Directions:

1. In a blender, combine the cream with the coconut milk, the walnuts and the other ingredients, pulse well, divide into cups and serve cold.

Nutrition:

calories 283, fat 11.8, fiber 0.3, carbs 4.7, protein 7.1

Chia & Coco Shake (vegan)

Preparation Time: 5 minutes

Cooking Time: 0 minute

Servings: 2

Ingredients:

- 1 tbsp. chia seeds
- 6 tbsp. water
- 1 cup full-fat coconut milk
- 2 tbsp. peanut butter (see recipe)
- 1 scoop organic soy protein powder (chocolate flavor)
- 1 tbsp. MCT oil (or coconut oil)
- Pinch of Himalayan salt
- 2-4 ice cubes or ½ cup of water

Directions:

1. Mix the chia seeds and 6 tablespoons of water in a small bowl; let sit for at least 30 minutes.
2. Transfer the soaked chia seeds and all other listed ingredients to a blender and blend for 2 minutes.

3. Transfer the shake to a large cup or shaker, serve, and enjoy!
4. Alternatively, store the smoothie in an airtight container or a mason jar, keep it in the fridge, and consume within 3 days.
5. Store for a maximum of 30 days in the freezer and thaw at room temperature.

Nutrition:

Calories: 509kcal, Net Carbs: 5.4g, Fat: 44.55g, Protein: 20.3g, Fiber: 7.45g, Sugar: 3.5g

NOTE

www.ingramcontent.com/pod-product-compliance
Lightning Source LLC
Chambersburg PA
CBHW070102120526
44589CB00033B/1509